What I Went Through

Shyness

Autism

Depression / Hating Myself

Being Unpopular

How I coped

Depression Cures

Schizophrenia Cure

Manic Depression Cure

Voices Cure

Imagining Pictures Making Faces

Worry

Crazy

Talking To The Psychiatrist

Making a decision

The Help I Got

Parents

Medication

Sexuality –Someone To Tell Me

Advice

Don't Sin All The Time

Don't Expect Fast Results

Affirmation

Find A Purpose In Life

Where I Went Wrong

Advice OnFriendship

Relationships With Girls

Some Advice

Suicide

Talking To The Samaritans

My Relationship with my parents

WHAT PARENTS SHOULD DO IN THEIR RELATIONSHIP WITH THEIR CHILD

WHAT I WENT THROUGH :

Shyness

I didn't know how to make friends : The simple the things – "I'm going to the soccer match do you want to come along". [see article on friendship]

When getting to know someone I never tried to develop the friendship early on – take risks which you need to do at the start to develop a friendship like saying "I'd like to visit your house" – that's a big plus when making a friend.

I didn't know how to hold a conversation : because I didn't realise that most people talk about ordinary things – like teachers / schools / homework / other friends / television.

The solution is not to go on a vast crash course memorising songs/ watching soaps – be true to yourself. You will find you can talk about the things that matter to you. It's okay to be different.. If you can accept your own opinions [you are accepting yourself] and others will accept you aswell.

Autism

Maybe you are someone who is autistic [you may not even realise you are] – you don't try to make friends but at the same time you like being near / in the company of others

– > in silence / not having to talk – that's okay too. Autism is not a cross it is a gift of peace / inner silence. Something I have learned about Autism – being with people – when they talk to you   – Autistic people feel under pressure to respond to talk back in the conversation – this is making the autistic person unhappy. What I have learned is tell the person who is Autistic just make a facial expression - smile; wink; nod your head in response to the person talking instead of talking back - you don't have to talk. Try out computers with autistic teenagers – they find it easier to express themselves in email format.

Depression / Hating myself

At first I used to get depressed everyday. It developed I became anti-social. I was fighting myself. I wouldn't let myself make friends. I found it difficult to make conversation. I withdrew into myself and daydreamed a lot. I kept running away from situations. I was prescribed medication but I kept giving it up and I needed to get medication that worked for me. I tried loads of self-help books but they didn't work because they didn't tell me about suffering - Where I Was At -> dealing with where I was right now. When I finally I did accept medication that works for me! My mind stabilised a lot. I learned ways of dealing with schizophrenia.

Being Unpopular

I know what it feels like to be unpopular – to have everyone talking about you and knowing everything about you. Does this mean your life is over. NO! Encourage your son to get involved in a hobby – join a cause : Like Greenpeace or Amnesty International or the youth wing of a political party. Your son is going to find a different class of people there and most probably will make friends there – [SHARED INTERESTS!!] You son can feel good if your son is doing good in the world – so get him involved in the soup kitchen; mentoring younger kids etc. Finally a relationship with God where your son talks to the Man Above every day about literally anything and everything in his life – Your son should make God his friend too.

HOW I COPED :

Depression Cures

Whenever you are depressed spend some time being silent within yourself for 5-25 minutes. You will feel a deep sense of peace afterwards - the more depressed you were the more peace you will feel after the silence. You may say it is too hard to maintain silence - the mind will wander - No! what you will find is that when you are depressed it is in this situation actually easy to be silent within yourself..
Another idea for curing depression is "Cant's". When you are depressed ask yourself what am I telling myself I can't do? Again you will find it easy to identify things that you are telling yourself you can't do [when you are depressed you are more in tune with yourself] Sometimes "Have to's" are the same as cant's. Again cant's are a cause of depression.
A fourth meal - People with depression fill themselves up with junk food - eat a fourth meal in the evening around 7/8 - proper food - food that you would eat at a meal if you are depressed - This also will help cure you of depression.
The last resort if you are still depressed after trying "cant's""four meals" and "silence" try enjoying yourself.

Schizophrenia Cure

If you suffer from schizophrenia - Just enjoy life and take your medication - in the long term [a few years] this will cure you and if depressed do as for depression.

Voices Cure

Sit at the opposite side to the door with your back against the wall on a chair – Stay there for 20 – 30 minutes. Focus on not talking – this works better than focusing on not thinking. The voices disappear – There is a psychological effect here – there is no one else in the room. Try to have noise down to a minimum.

Imagining Pictures making faces

If you look at a picture of a person / religious image and it seems to be making faces at you. Say hi to the picture by name if possible this is a cure for this. Pictures stop making faces at you.

Worry

Don't judge a person by their facial expression. I used to worry over my dad – looking at his facial expression which could be negative but each time he was okay. Instead judge a person by the sound of their voice – that is how to know if someone needs help or not. Another idea – if someone is worried –don't worry back. Two other ways to deal with worry are 1. Be tough and choose to hold firm and 2. Every time you are about to worry yawn – keep doing this – it may take several minutes where you start and stop worrying so you will need to yawn several times but it does get rid of the worry feeling eventually

Crazy

Try this out – for someone in the midst of a nervous breakdown – They need noise – lots of this – It straightens out their thinking. I know what it is like to think crazy thoughtS – I had a nervous breakdown myself – It will be obvious to the parents that a teenager was not acting right for several days. – The basic thing with a nervous breakdown is the person's ability to say "no" gets severely damaged – they come up with crazy ideas and are unable to say no to them. During my breakdown – my parents brought me to the local doctor [GP] who recommended a good psychiatrist to them [this is the approach I recommend you take].

Talking to the Psychiatrist

I wasn't very intelligent when I visited the psychiatrist. She would ask me questions [she was perceptive] but I was not able to answer | unable to think clearly. However she proscribed some very good medication for me which did over a few months improve my health. It was she who told me I has heterosexual. She would ask me questions but I never prepared for any meeting in advance – to organize my thoughts. I also never put into practice any of the suggestions she made. Psychiatrists can and would love to talk to parents of the mentally ill son. Eventually I left her in the lurch and just chose no longer to attend [this does happen in several cases]. My health slowly but surely deteriorated after leaving her. I could have made far more progress with my psychiatrist if I had prepared for her meetings a point I recommend you stress to your teenager.

Making a decision

Repeat the following "Yes, No, Yes, No, Yes, No, Yes, Yes. Another strategy is the following if they ask you a question repeat the question back to them.

THE HELP I GOT :.

Parents

They got me to a day hospital where I could meet with a doctor and receive medication. They didn't pressuriseme into talking to them they trusted I would talk to the doctor. They made sure I took my medication. They loved me which is all they can do, through my suffering and in the long run I benefited from their constant love and encouragement. People find it easier to talk to a doctor that their parents. Don't force your child to talk to you.

Medication

At first I got medication that didn't work properly for me. Eventually I got the right sort of medication. It helped me think straight and you didn't realise you were not alright before getting the medication. I needed to be taking it for a while to say I am truly level-headed and to say this is the way I should be. I don't get crazy thoughts when I stick to the medication. I have a level of self-esteem / I can do more things. I went through the ususal – lapses in taking medication – the ususal excuses people with depression come up with "side affects". The reality is these days most medications are pretty good with only basic side affects.

Sexuality – Someone to tell me

I needed someone to tell about my sexuality someone I trusted and looked up to. I always had difficulty with my sexuality – what was acceptable. I was heterosexual but autistic and schizophrenic to boot all in the one. You need to tell your son – noticing a girls breasts is not a sin [you can think about it but try not to dwell on it] They may get slightly aroused when they look at a beautiful girl tell them again this is perfectly natural [again you can think about it but try not to dwell on it]. Self-control is important too – if your son is too distracted tell them to think about interesting things – "whose at the top of the league in baseball; when does Liverpool play man united; What chance has Tiger Woods of making a comeback."

ADVICE :

Don't sin all the time

Refuse to sin. There are situations where you might find if you tell something you will suffer but you would be surprised because usually you don't. Not sinning is good for your self-esteem. It forces you to think. No matter what the circumstances refuse to sin. People in this world put a priority on feelings – No! feelings come second – Refusing to sin comes first – it makes for stronger happier people. You have to remain constantly vigilant when it comes to your ego – your ego should only be as high as you are. Another point is that you have privacy rights – you are not forced to tell people private things about yourself. Refusing to sin boosts your self-esteem.

Don't expect fast results

Suffering is not going to go away in a day or a week no matter what you do. I know you don't like suffering but that does not mean that you cannot have self-esteem and feel good about yourself even while you are going through tough times.

Affirmation

"I am worthy of love" – stick to this affirmation – It's probably the best affirmation I have ever heard. Raise your right arm fist closed and say any affirmation you want – using this method is ten times stronger than any verbal affirmation. Another idea is at the end of every day to list all the good things that happened to you that day.

Find a purpose in life

If you are cured of depression I don't just want you to live an ordinary life I want you to become a force for good in the world. Counsellors, psychiatrists etc. please work with your patients and find a cause / purpose for them in life.

Religion

I am putting this in man – you must have a relationship with Jesus or Mohammed and GOD– THAT MEANS PRAYER! There is no other rock on which you can always depend on. You gotta pray no matter how you feel.

Start Small

You gotta learn this in life – wherever you are; whatever you are doing – start small – don't take on loads of things; don't try to make loads of friends all at once; don't be too ambitious.

Bedroom

Get out of the bedroom – bedrooms are for sleeping in – not for working in.

Silence

There is too much noise in this world – It is suffocating your soul. Silence brings you closer to God – God communicates to person in silence. Silence makes a person more intelligent – noise does the opposite. Go to church or something during the day [not during a mass] – spend a few minutes in the silence of the church. Alternatively spend five minutes just sitting with your eyes closed in silence.

Taking Care of yourself

My mantra for taking care of yourself = warm / soft / dry. Surround yourself with happy things – happy music; happy television programmes; a happy book. A way of relaxing is to wear your pajamas during the day while you are in the house it has the effect of relaxing you.

Suffering

When you are really suffering keep yourself busy

Hope

Keep trying even if things look grim – things do get better. There is such a thing as an "Afterwards" even if you fail – your efforts are building a future after the failure.

Love

Notice the things they like. You want the other person to feel loved that's the mantra. Don't try to please people – people respect honesty. When someone shows you something they are doing – they are looking for appreciation / interest. Some teenagers are too used to saying no to one of their parents –get them to listen and accept what this parent is saying because a lot of the time they are right. Your child will realize this.

Four Bases

You may feel depressed or stressed – To handle these stresses – there are four bases – Rest / Work / Pray / Enjoy. If your self-esteem is pretty low then enjoy yourself. If your faith is weak pray. Pope John Paul II once said that all of us at some stages in our life need an extended period of rest. If you are not stressed and you are not feeling spiritually weak then work is the answer,.

WHERE I WENT WRONG :

I didn't stick to things

I started things like scouts, or a job or yoga and gave them up. I started a particular affirmation but after 3 /4 weeks I stopped using them.

I wouldn't fight

When people started saying things about me I didn't speak up for myself. I felt it was wrong to criticise the other person. I avoided people. I didn't hang on to my friends. I let them walk all over me. I kept running away.

I said I can't because too often…

I said I can't make friends with such and such a person because my enemies might talk to them and turn them against me. Stand up for yourself!
I said I can't go out with someone because I have no friends – yes you can they are interested in you.

I wouldn't take medication which I needed

I felt taking medication was unhealthy / I felt I didn't need it. I didn't realise I wasn't thinking straight. I kept stopping taking my medications. Now I take medication without thinking twice just like eating food and I know it is good for me too.

I worked too hard

I was doing all honours subjects at school. I was working long hours with virtually no social life, no time to relax each day and socialise / watch tv. It never occurred to me that I should ease up and tell my teachers I was working too hard and needed to do pass level in a few subjects. For me English was the subject that was taking up most of my time at home. You'd be surprised where people end up. People with degrees ending up in mediocre jobs and people with certs.ending up running their own businesses. You don't need to go to University to get a qualification you can go to an [I.T.] / private college.where the qualifications are just as good but the entry requirements are lower. Working too hard was damaging my mental health seriously. You need to take care of yourself. You should be able to relax for at least an hour before you go to bed each night.

ADVICE ON FRIENDSHIP :

Do not pick someone and then try to be their friend; instead be friendly with everyone and let friendships happen over time.

If you are in a room with two or more people that you are being friendly with do not feel you have to talk to / say hello to all of them; instead talk to / say hello to whoever / how many people you feel like at the time.

Do not worry if someone frowns / be's jealous for you not talking to them, peoples opinions of you usually change with each encounter until you have made solid friends.

Do not judge by appearances / dislike someone instead say to yourself "I do not know this person well" because in all probability if you got to know them, over time you might like them.

A simple hand-wave, smile or hello is enough to start off with when being friendly with everyone.

Do not worry as long as everyone see's you doing it you will be able to let friendships happen instead of being put in difficult situations.

Do not try to hide your emotions if you are depressed say so.

You can be friends with whoever you want.

RELATIONSHIPS WITH GIRLS :

I was the shy, polite nice guy – always saying yes to everyone's request. A lot of women fall for that kind of guy – TROUBLE : for someone who had no self-confidence. I was terrified of women – I lacked all self-confidence in relating to them. But I actually did fall in love with someone and when I did I felt full of self-confidence.

SOME ADVICE

Don't make direct eye-contact with women this is an attraction
generator unless of course you want to go out with them
In college : say firmly in full hearing of other female students and male
students "I am definitely not going out with anyone in first year"– Going
out with someone in first year can prove to be a big headache when you
break off and people start fighting over whose friends are whose
When you are in love – the best way to be in love is where you have
both got to know each other first. You feel like you can talk about
anything even personal secrets. You don't struggle to come up with
ideas about what to talk about [socializing usually a difficulty for people
with schizophrenia]. You accept the other person totally and are relaxed
around them. Falling in love is good medicine for people with
schizophrenia. All your fears of [no confidence | not knowing what to
say | what to do with each other which in my case I have felt at times –
expecting that this would always be the case]
If your son wants to find a girlfriend – I encourage him to make friends
first with girls – FRIENDS NO COMMITMENTS ! Some girls get on better
with men and are more open to friendships with boys even hanging out
with them – So the advice I would give your son is to befriend this kind
of girl.

SUICIDE :

A lot of teenagers with Schizophrenia make an attempt at suicide –
tablets is the most obvious way. I have tried a few times for various

reasons – I will give two examples one was where I was being gossiped a lot and talked a lot about – I refused to accept the situation so I made a half-botched attempt at suicide using a blade to my Kneck [it did not work] This was a protest. I didn't see that life changes – people change – situations change – That there are always opportunities coming up in life. I didn't think past the present moment I was in – it was a very specific moment. The second attempt was more serious this was an attempt based on me feeling very withdrawn. I took some tablets this time not enough [not enough is a common occurrence in suicide attempts] – I acted quickly. In this situation the teenager needs to be hospitalised. It would be a good thing if your teenager had a mobile phone of their own and was aware of telephone numbers they could ring where they could talk in confidence to someone. In either case you must bring your child straight to the doctor where he will assess him.

[For Ireland And The UK]

TALKING TO THE SAMARITANS :

Do not be afraid to talk to the Samaritans. I have done so myself. I have had a tough time. When I went to the Samaritans I was put at ease almost immediately. They made me feel like I was in control again. They did not force me to talk and I did not feel that I had to talk. Even if you only tell them something general which is your freedom to do so – It is still worth a visit. If you are the kind of person who is trying to change their life for the better but has not succeeded so far – I would recommend a visit to the Samaritans. Do not wait until you are very depressed. Do not feel you have to be very depressed to visit them. I found talking to the Samaritans a positive experience. They will not judge you no matter what you tell them.

Finally if you are on medication stay on it – I need medication myself for depression at least until I have been feeling well for a few years and then I would be taken off medication very slowly

MY RELATIONSHIP WITH MY PARENTS

First my Dad – During my teenage years I had a lot of difficulty with my dad. My dad is a person who likes DIY and would regularly recruit me into working with him. I had schizophrenia and Autism at the same time – Which meant I really could not handle my dad's desire to ask me questions. I always felt negatively to him back then – And always felt guilty if I refused to work with him. Now I have a great relationship with

my dad. I had to be proactive about my relationship with my dad – I started affirming that he was a good man [Which he was] frequently. My love for him blossomed. I got stuck into working with him – To be frank I was just bone lazy back then. I learned that my dad's opinion was

the right one. Right now in society – teenagers are just bone lazy to be honest – but as a person grows – family members turn back to their parents and depend on them. In the bible it says – Honour your father and your mother. I have regrets in my life with my relationship with my dad [I should have realised that my dad wanted the best for me] He was leading me on the right course – I just was too young to realise this. Don't make the mistakes I made – work with your dad and affirm him as

a good man and that instead of refusing to listen to what he said and just saying no to him all the time; I should have loved my dad more. Now my dad is my favorite person along with my mum. Mum did something properly back then – She did not force me to talk – She would quite happily sit in silence in the room. And children are more inclined to talk and approach the silent parent.

WHAT PARENTS SHOULD DO IN THEIR RELATIONSHIP WITH THEIR CHILD

There is an old Irish saying –   "Praise The Youth And The Will Follow". Children can get very low self-esteem in a difficult relationship with their parents – Have someone approach them ask them "Do you like ice cream"; "Do you like toast? Etc. Get them to think in terms of things they like doing. If a child asks permission for something say yes sometimes and no other times – Encourage them to realise they will not always get their way in life – but not to give up asking for things. Children are very impressionable and childhood decisions or experiences can have a profound and life-time affect on them. An example from me – My parents sent me to my room for misbehaviour. As I sat in my room I suddenly thought – maybe this is my fault. And for years into my life including my adult life I kept taking the blame for everything

THANK YOU FOR READING THIS BOOK

GOD BLESS AND PEACE BE WITH YOU
PAUL ARMSTRONG

P.S. IF YOU WOULD LIKE TO MAKE ANY COMMENTS ON THIS EBOOK
YOU MAY CONTACT ME AT armstrop76@gmail.com

P.P.S STICK WITH THE MEDICATION!!